# HEALTHY

# MEDITERRANEAN DIET

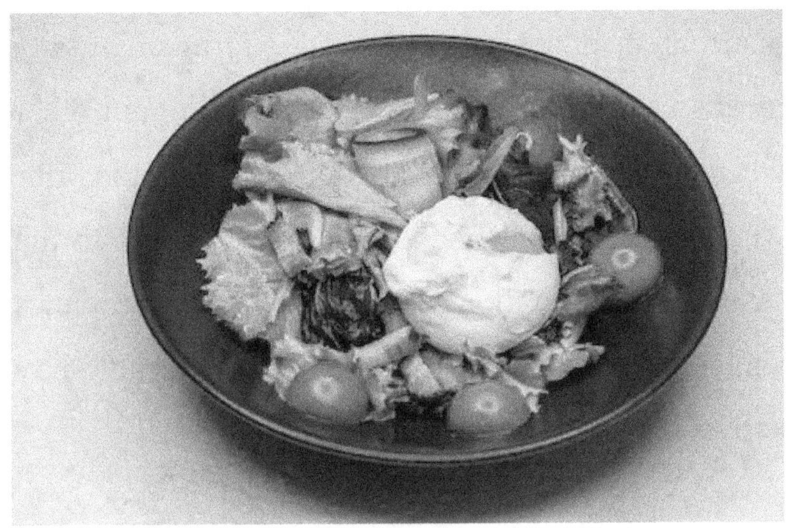

*20 Healthy Recipes*

## Wilbert M. Jensen

**CHECK MY OTHER BOOKS HERE**

# TABLE OF CONTENT

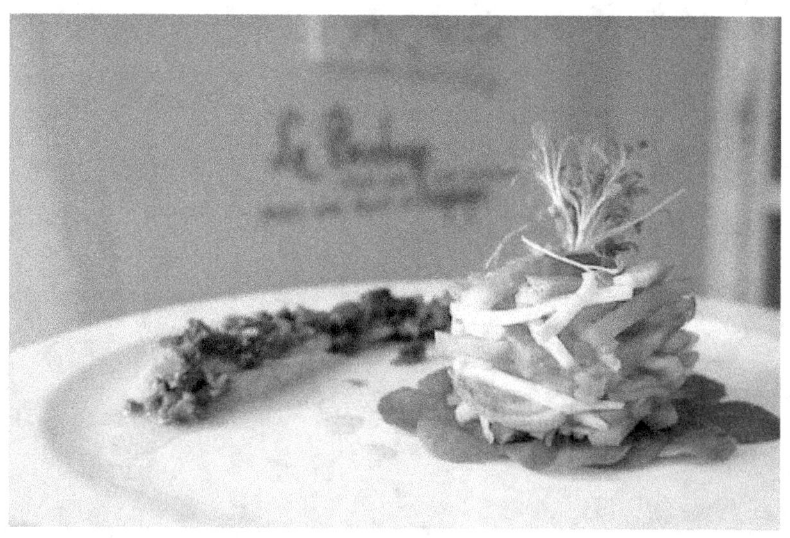

# INTRODUCTION

Solomon embraced the secrets of longevity buried in the Mediterranean wind in the sun-kissed hamlet of Santorini. His days were a symphony of olives, tomatoes, and fresh herbs.

He nurtured a garden with aged hands, where vivid veggies grew in the Aegean light. Solomon, a model of health, enthusiastically adopted the heart-healthy Mediterranean diet.

His dinners were a kaleidoscope of grilled fish drizzled with olive oil and served with crisp greens. Each bite was a celebration of life, a ballet of tastes that whispered the stories of previous generations.

Solomon's vigor became a monument to the Mediterranean diet's replenishing effect. He stood as a living representation of a culture that cherished nutritious food and the delight of shared, healthful meals as laughter resonated through his vine-covered patio. Solomon's legacy echoed through the cobblestone walkways, a testament to the ageless harmony found at the core of Mediterranean living.

# DELICIOUS HEALTHY MEDITERRANEAN DIET RECIPES

## Greek Salad

**Ingredients:**

2 large tomatoes, diced

1 cucumber, sliced

1 red onion, thinly sliced

1 cup Kalamata olives, pitted

200g feta cheese, crumbled

2 tbsp extra virgin olive oil

1 tbsp red wine vinegar

Salt and pepper to taste

**Preparation:**

Combine tomatoes, cucumber, red onion, and olives in a bowl.

Drizzle with olive oil and red wine vinegar.

Add feta cheese and season with salt and pepper. Toss gently.

## Grilled Lemon Garlic Chicken

**Ingredients:**

4 boneless, skinless chicken breasts

3 tbsp olive oil

3 cloves garlic, minced

1 lemon, juiced

1 tsp dried oregano

Salt and pepper to taste

**Preparation:**

In a bowl, mix olive oil, minced garlic, lemon juice, oregano, salt, and pepper.

Marinate chicken in the mixture for 30 minutes.

Grill until fully cooked, approximately 6-8 minutes per side.

## Mediterranean Quinoa Bowl

**Ingredients:**

1 cup quinoa, rinsed

2 cups water

1 cup cherry tomatoes, halved

1 cucumber, diced

1/2 cup black olives, sliced

1/4 cup feta cheese, crumbled

2 tbsp olive oil

1 tbsp balsamic vinegar

**Preparation:**

Cook quinoa according to package instructions.

Mix quinoa with tomatoes, cucumber, olives, and feta.

Drizzle with olive oil and balsamic vinegar. Toss gently.

## Mediterranean Roasted Vegetables

**Ingredients:**

1 zucchini, sliced

1 eggplant, diced

1 red bell pepper, sliced

1 yellow bell pepper, sliced

1 red onion, sliced

3 tbsp olive oil

1 tsp dried thyme

Salt and pepper to taste

**Preparation:**

Preheat oven to 400°F (200°C).

Toss vegetables with olive oil, thyme, salt, and pepper.

Roast for 25-30 minutes or until vegetables are tender.

## Lemon Garlic Shrimp Pasta

**Ingredients:**

8 oz whole wheat spaghetti

1 lb shrimp, peeled and deveined

3 tbsp olive oil

4 cloves garlic, minced

1 lemon, zest and juice

1/4 cup fresh parsley, chopped

Salt and pepper to taste

**Preparation:**

Cook spaghetti according to package instructions.

In a pan, sauté shrimp in olive oil and garlic until cooked.

Toss cooked spaghetti with shrimp, lemon zest, lemon juice, parsley, salt, and pepper.

Feel free to adjust portion sizes and ingredients based on personal preferences and dietary needs. Enjoy your delicious and nutritious Mediterranean meals!

## Mediterranean Stuffed Bell Peppers

**Ingredients:**

4 large bell peppers, halved and seeds removed

1 cup cooked quinoa

1 can (15 oz) chickpeas, drained and rinsed

1 cup cherry tomatoes, diced

1/2 cup feta cheese, crumbled

2 tbsp olive oil

1 tsp dried oregano

Salt and pepper to taste

**Preparation:**

Preheat oven to 375°F (190°C).

In a bowl, mix quinoa, chickpeas, tomatoes, feta, olive oil, oregano, salt, and pepper.

Stuff bell peppers with the mixture and bake for 25-30 minutes.

## Mediterranean Hummus Wrap

**Ingredients:**

Whole wheat tortillas

1 cup hummus

1 cup baby spinach

1 cucumber, julienned

1/2 cup cherry tomatoes, halved

1/4 cup red onion, thinly sliced

Kalamata olives, sliced (optional)

**Preparation:**

Spread hummus on each tortilla.

Layer with spinach, cucumber, tomatoes, red onion, and olives.

Roll up tightly and slice in half.

## Mediterranean Lentil Soup

**Ingredients:**

1 cup dried lentils, rinsed

1 onion, chopped

2 carrots, diced

2 celery stalks, chopped

3 cloves garlic, minced

1 can (14 oz) diced tomatoes

6 cups vegetable broth

1 tsp ground cumin

1 tsp dried thyme

Salt and pepper to taste

**Preparation:**

In a pot, sauté onion, carrots, celery, and garlic until softened.

Add lentils, tomatoes, vegetable broth, cumin, thyme, salt, and pepper. Simmer for 25-30 minutes.

## Mediterranean Baked Salmon

**Ingredients:**

4 salmon fillets

2 tbsp olive oil

2 tbsp lemon juice

1 tsp dried oregano

1 tsp garlic powder

Salt and pepper to taste

**Preparation:**

Preheat oven to 400°F (200°C).

Place salmon fillets on a baking sheet.

Mix olive oil, lemon juice, oregano, garlic powder, salt, and pepper. Brush over salmon.

Bake for 15-20 minutes or until salmon is cooked through.

## Mediterranean Chickpea Salad

Ingredients:

2 cans (15 oz each) chickpeas, drained and rinsed

1 cucumber, diced

1 cup cherry tomatoes, halved

1/2 red onion, finely chopped

1/4 cup fresh parsley, chopped

3 tbsp olive oil

2 tbsp red wine vinegar

1 tsp dried oregano

Salt and pepper to taste

**Preparation:**

In a large bowl, combine chickpeas, cucumber, tomatoes, red onion, and parsley.

Whisk together olive oil, red wine vinegar, oregano, salt, and pepper. Pour over the salad and toss gently.

# Mediterranean Eggplant Dip (Baba Ganoush)

**Ingredients:**

2 large eggplants

2 cloves garlic, minced

3 tbsp tahini

2 tbsp lemon juice

2 tbsp olive oil

1/4 cup fresh parsley, chopped

Salt and pepper to taste

**Preparation:**

Preheat oven to 400°F (200°C).

Roast whole eggplants in the oven for 40-45 minutes until skin is charred.

Peel eggplants, mash the flesh, and mix with garlic, tahini, lemon juice, olive oil, parsley, salt, and pepper.

## Mediterranean Whole Wheat Pita Pizza

**Ingredients:**

Whole wheat pita bread

1/2 cup hummus

1 cup baby spinach

1/2 cup cherry tomatoes, sliced

1/4 cup black olives, sliced

1/4 cup feta cheese, crumbled

Olive oil for drizzling

**Preparation:**

Preheat oven to 375°F (190°C).

Spread hummus on pita bread, layer with spinach, tomatoes, olives, and feta.

Drizzle with olive oil and bake for 10-12 minutes.

## Mediterranean Tzatziki Sauce

**Ingredients:**

1 cup Greek yogurt

1 cucumber, finely grated

2 cloves garlic, minced

1 tbsp fresh dill, chopped

1 tbsp olive oil

Salt and pepper to taste

**Preparation:**

Mix Greek yogurt, grated cucumber, garlic, dill, olive oil, salt, and pepper in a bowl.

Refrigerate for at least 30 minutes before serving.

# Mediterranean Stuffed Grape Leaves (Dolma)

**Ingredients:**

1 jar grape leaves, drained

1 cup cooked white rice

1/2 cup pine nuts, toasted

1/4 cup fresh mint, chopped

1/4 cup fresh parsley, chopped

2 tbsp olive oil

1 lemon, juiced

Salt and pepper to taste

**Preparation:**

Mix rice, pine nuts, mint, parsley, olive oil, lemon juice, salt, and pepper in a bowl.

Place a spoonful of the mixture onto each grape leaf, fold, and roll tightly.

**Mediterranean Chickpea and Spinach Stew**

**Ingredients:**

2 cans (15 oz each) chickpeas, drained and rinsed

1 onion, chopped

3 cloves garlic, minced

1 can (14 oz) diced tomatoes

4 cups baby spinach

2 tbsp olive oil

1 tsp cumin

1 tsp paprika

Salt and pepper to taste

**Preparation:**

Sauté onion and garlic in olive oil until softened.

Add chickpeas, tomatoes, spinach, cumin, paprika, salt, and pepper. Simmer for 15-20 minutes.

## Mediterranean Roasted Red Pepper Hummus

**Ingredients:**

1 can (15 oz) chickpeas, drained and rinsed

2 large roasted red peppers, peeled and chopped

3 tbsp tahini

2 cloves garlic, minced

2 tbsp lemon juice

2 tbsp olive oil

1 tsp ground cumin

Salt and pepper to taste

**Preparation:**

In a food processor, blend chickpeas, roasted red peppers, tahini, garlic, lemon juice, olive oil, cumin, salt, and pepper until smooth.

## Mediterranean Orzo Salad

**Ingredients:**

1 cup orzo pasta, cooked

1 cup cherry tomatoes, halved

1/2 cucumber, diced

1/4 cup red onion, finely chopped

1/4 cup feta cheese, crumbled

2 tbsp olive oil

1 tbsp red wine vinegar

1 tsp dried oregano

Salt and pepper to taste

**Preparation:**

In a bowl, combine orzo, tomatoes, cucumber, red onion, and feta.

Drizzle with olive oil, red wine vinegar, oregano, salt, and pepper. Toss gently.

## Mediterranean Grilled Vegetable Wrap

**Ingredients:**

Whole wheat wraps

1 zucchini, sliced

1 eggplant, sliced

1 red bell pepper, sliced

1 yellow bell pepper, sliced

2 tbsp olive oil

1 tsp dried thyme

Hummus for spreading

**Preparation:**

Toss zucchini, eggplant, and bell peppers with olive oil and thyme.

Grill vegetables until tender.

Spread hummus on wraps, add grilled vegetables, and roll up.

## Mediterranean Baked Falafel

**Ingredients:**

2 cans (15 oz each) chickpeas, drained and rinsed

1/2 cup fresh parsley, chopped

1/4 cup red onion, chopped

2 cloves garlic, minced

1 tsp ground cumin

1 tsp ground coriander

1/2 cup whole wheat breadcrumbs

Olive oil for brushing

Preparation:

Preheat oven to 375°F (190°C).

In a food processor, blend chickpeas, parsley, red onion, garlic, cumin, coriander, and breadcrumbs until mixture holds together.

Form into small patties, brush with olive oil, and bake for 20-25 minutes.

## Mediterranean Yogurt Parfait

**Ingredients:**

1 cup Greek yogurt

1 cup mixed berries (strawberries, blueberries, raspberries)

1/4 cup granola

2 tbsp honey

**Preparation:**

In a glass, layer Greek yogurt, mixed berries, and granola.

Drizzle with honey before serving.

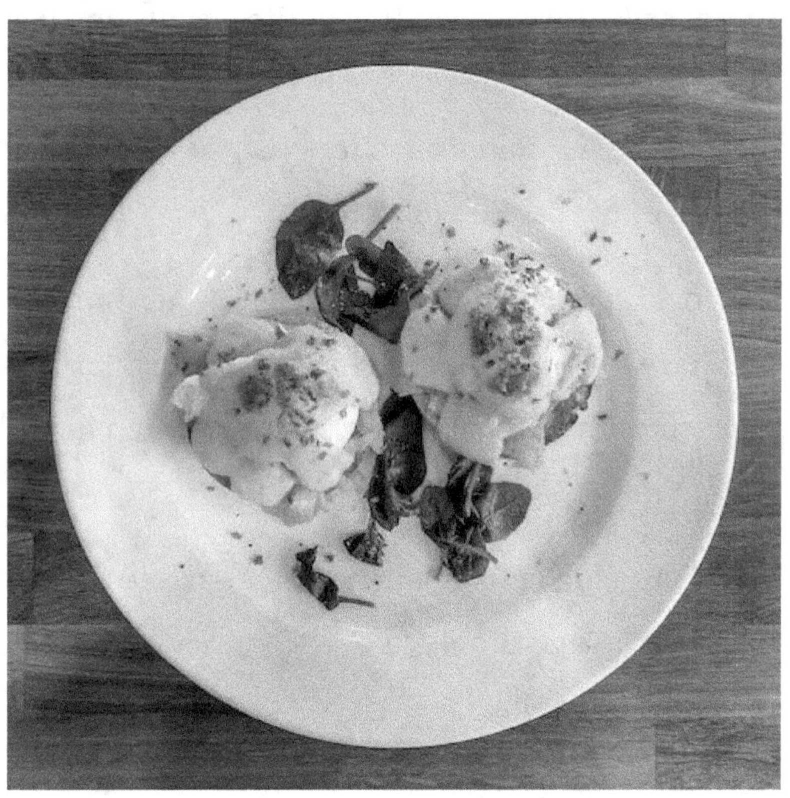

# CONCLUSION

Each recipe in the Healthy Mediterranean Recipes Cookbook's symphony of flavors is a tribute to the art of nourishing both the body and the spirit.

These meals are a celebration of life, health, and the intimate relationship between culture and food, from the vivid colors of Greek salads to the rich fragrances of roasted vegetables.

The cookbook echoes the knowledge of generations who have embraced the Mediterranean way of life via each carefully picked ingredient and step in the preparation.

Allow this collection to serve as a compass to guide you on a voyage of wholesome living, where tasty and nutritious collide.

May each mouthful serve as a reminder that the simplicity of a well-balanced meal provides not only nutrition but also the way to a robust and